THE SUGAR-DETOX COOKBOOK FOR SENIORS

2024

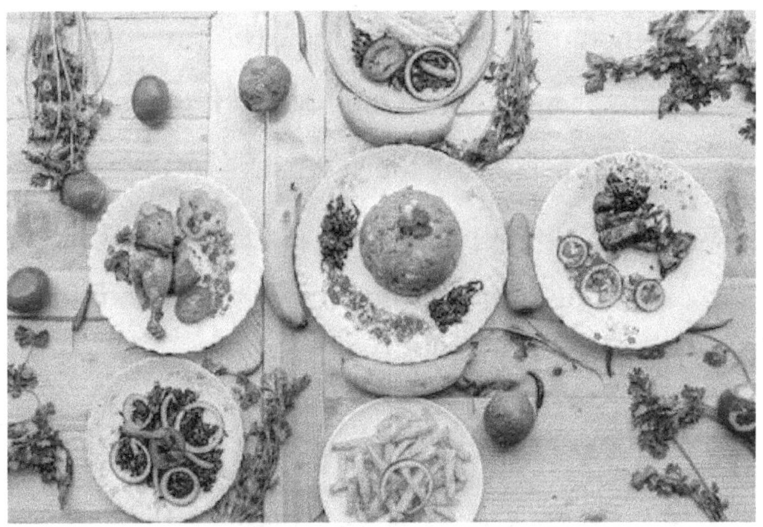

Over 20 Recipes for All Program Levels

Wilbert M. Jensen

Copyright © 2024 by Wilbert M. Jensen

All rights reserved.

GAIN ACCESS TO MORE BOOKS FROM ME

TABLE OF CONTENT

INTRODUCTION

Abby, a vivacious senior with a sweet appetite, was at a crossroads when her doctor suggested a sugar detox for improved health. Determined to make a good difference, she discovered the "Sweet Liberation" cookbook for seniors. Abby was astounded by the delectable dishes that promised guilt-free enjoyment as she flipped through the pages.

Abby set off on her sugar-free quest, armed with her newly acquired culinary talents. The cookbook became her reliable friend, guiding her through creative meals that substituted refined sweets with healthier alternatives.

Soon, Abby's kitchen was filled with the perfume of sugar-free treats, and her energy levels skyrocketed. With each tasty meal, Abby not only adopted a better lifestyle, but also inspired her fellow seniors.

The "Sweet Liberation" cookbook not only changed her diet, but it also filled her senior years with renewed health and enthusiasm for life.

DELICIOUS THE SUGAR DETOX COOKBOOK FOR SENIORS RECIPES

Berry Bliss Smoothie:

Ingredients:

1 cup mixed berries (strawberries, blueberries, raspberries)

1/2 banana

1 cup unsweetened almond milk

1 tablespoon chia seeds

Preparation:

Blend all ingredients until smooth.

Zesty Avocado Salad:

Ingredients:

1 ripe avocado, diced

1 cup cherry tomatoes, halved

1 cucumber, diced

2 tablespoons olive oil

1 tablespoon lemon juice

Preparation:

Toss all ingredients in a bowl, drizzle with olive oil and lemon juice.

Cauliflower Rice Stir-Fry:

Ingredients:

2 cups cauliflower rice

1 cup mixed vegetables (bell peppers, broccoli, carrots)

2 tablespoons low-sodium soy sauce

1 tablespoon olive oil

Preparation:

Sauté vegetables in olive oil, add cauliflower rice, stir in soy sauce.

Lemon Herb Baked Chicken:

Ingredients:

4 boneless, skinless chicken breasts

2 tablespoons fresh lemon juice

1 teaspoon dried thyme

1 teaspoon garlic powder

Preparation:

Marinate chicken with lemon juice, thyme, and garlic powder; bake until cooked.

Green Goddess Soup:

Ingredients:

2 cups spinach

1 cup kale

1 onion, chopped

2 cloves garlic, minced

4 cups vegetable broth

Preparation:

Sauté onion and garlic, add greens and broth, simmer until vegetables are tender.

Salmon with Dill Sauce:

Ingredients:

4 salmon fillets

2 tablespoons fresh dill, chopped

1 tablespoon Dijon mustard

1 tablespoon olive oil

Preparation:

Mix dill, mustard, and olive oil; brush on salmon, bake until flaky.

Quinoa-Stuffed Bell Peppers:

Ingredients:

4 bell peppers, halved

1 cup cooked quinoa

1 cup black beans, drained

1 cup diced tomatoes

Preparation:

Mix quinoa, beans, and tomatoes; stuff into peppers, bake until peppers are tender.

Cinnamon Baked Apples:

Ingredients:

4 apples, cored and sliced

1 teaspoon cinnamon

1 tablespoon coconut oil

1 tablespoon chopped nuts (optional)

Preparation:

Toss apples with cinnamon and coconut oil; bake until tender, sprinkle with nuts.

Turmeric-Ginger Carrot Soup:

Ingredients:

4 cups carrots, chopped

1 tablespoon fresh ginger, grated

1 teaspoon ground turmeric

4 cups vegetable broth

Preparation:

Cook carrots, ginger, and turmeric in broth, blend until smooth.

Mango Lime Salsa Chicken:

Ingredients:

4 boneless, skinless chicken thighs

1 mango, diced

1 lime, juiced

2 tablespoons cilantro, chopped

Preparation:

Grill or bake chicken, top with mango-lime salsa and cilantro.

Greek Salad with Tzatziki Dressing:

Ingredients:

2 cups cucumber, diced

1 cup cherry tomatoes, halved

1/2 cup feta cheese, crumbled

1/4 cup Greek yogurt

1 tablespoon fresh dill, chopped

Preparation:

Combine cucumber, tomatoes, and feta; mix Greek yogurt and dill for dressing.

Cabbage and Mushroom Stir-Fry:

Ingredients:

2 cups cabbage, shredded

1 cup mushrooms, sliced

2 tablespoons soy sauce

1 tablespoon sesame oil

Preparation:

Sauté cabbage and mushrooms in sesame oil, stir in soy sauce.

Baked Pears with Walnuts:

Ingredients:

4 ripe pears, halved

1/2 cup walnuts, chopped

1 teaspoon cinnamon

1 tablespoon honey (optional)

Preparation:

Place pears on a baking sheet, sprinkle with walnuts and cinnamon; drizzle with honey if desired.

Spinach and Artichoke Stuffed Chicken:

Ingredients:

4 boneless, skinless chicken breasts

1 cup spinach, chopped

1/2 cup artichoke hearts, chopped

1/4 cup Parmesan cheese, grated

Preparation:

Mix spinach, artichoke, and Parmesan; stuff into chicken, bake until cooked through.

Sesame Ginger Salmon Patties:

Ingredients:

2 cans (14 oz each) salmon, drained

2 tablespoons soy sauce

1 tablespoon sesame oil

1 teaspoon fresh ginger, grated

Preparation:

Combine salmon, soy sauce, sesame oil, and ginger; form into patties, pan-fry until golden.

Cucumber Noodle Salad with Mint:

Ingredients:

2 large cucumbers, spiralized

1 cup cherry tomatoes, halved

1/4 cup fresh mint, chopped

2 tablespoons olive oil

Preparation:

Toss cucumber noodles, tomatoes, and mint with olive oil.

Lemon Herb Roasted Veggies:

Ingredients:

4 cups mixed vegetables (zucchini, bell peppers, carrots)

2 tablespoons olive oil

1 tablespoon fresh lemon juice

1 teaspoon dried herbs (rosemary, thyme)

Preparation:

Toss vegetables in olive oil, lemon juice, and herbs; roast until golden.

Blueberry Chia Seed Pudding:

Ingredients:

1 cup almond milk

1/2 cup chia seeds

1 cup blueberries

1 teaspoon vanilla extract

Preparation:

Mix almond milk, chia seeds, blueberries, and vanilla extract; refrigerate until pudding-like consistency.

Stuffed Bell Peppers with Turkey and Quinoa:

Ingredients:

4 bell peppers, halved

1 cup cooked quinoa

1/2 lb lean ground turkey, cooked

1 cup tomato sauce

Preparation:

Mix quinoa, turkey, and half of the tomato sauce; stuff into peppers, top with remaining sauce, bake until peppers are tender.

Coconut Almond Energy Bites:

Ingredients:

1 cup unsweetened shredded coconut

1/2 cup almond butter

1/4 cup honey

1 teaspoon vanilla extract

Preparation:

Combine coconut, almond butter, honey, and vanilla; shape into small bites, refrigerate until firm.

MEAL PLAN

Day 1:

Breakfast: Berry Bliss Smoothie

Ingredients: Mixed berries, banana, unsweetened almond milk, chia seeds.

Preparation: Blend all ingredients until smooth.

Lunch: Zesty Avocado Salad

Ingredients: Ripe avocado, cherry tomatoes, cucumber, olive oil, lemon juice.

Preparation: Toss ingredients in a bowl, drizzle with olive oil and lemon juice.

Dinner: Cauliflower Rice Stir-Fry

Ingredients: Cauliflower rice, mixed vegetables, low-sodium soy sauce, olive oil.

Preparation: Sauté vegetables in olive oil, add cauliflower rice, stir in soy sauce.

Day 2:

Breakfast: Lemon Herb Baked Chicken

Ingredients: Boneless, skinless chicken breasts, fresh lemon juice, dried thyme, garlic powder.

Preparation: Marinate chicken; bake until cooked.

Lunch: Green Goddess Soup

Ingredients: Spinach, kale, onion, garlic, vegetable broth.

Preparation: Sauté onion and garlic, add greens and broth, simmer until tender.

Dinner: Salmon with Dill Sauce

Ingredients: Salmon fillets, fresh dill, Dijon mustard, olive oil.

Preparation: Mix dill, mustard, and olive oil; brush on salmon, bake until flaky.

Day 3:

Breakfast: Quinoa-Stuffed Bell Peppers

Ingredients: Bell peppers, cooked quinoa, black beans, diced tomatoes.

Preparation: Mix quinoa, beans, and tomatoes; stuff into peppers, bake until tender.

Lunch: Cinnamon Baked Apples

Ingredients: Apples, cinnamon, coconut oil, chopped nuts (optional).

Preparation: Toss apples with cinnamon and coconut oil; bake until tender.

Dinner: Turmeric-Ginger Carrot Soup

Ingredients: Carrots, fresh ginger, ground turmeric, vegetable broth.

Preparation: Cook carrots, ginger, and turmeric in broth, blend until smooth.

Day 4:

Breakfast: Mango Lime Salsa Chicken

Ingredients: Boneless, skinless chicken thighs, mango, lime, cilantro.

Preparation: Grill or bake chicken, top with mango-lime salsa and cilantro.

Lunch: Greek Salad with Tzatziki Dressing

Ingredients: Cucumber, cherry tomatoes, feta cheese, Greek yogurt, fresh dill.

Preparation: Combine cucumber, tomatoes, and feta; mix Greek yogurt and dill for dressing.

Dinner: Cabbage and Mushroom Stir-Fry

Ingredients: Cabbage, mushrooms, soy sauce, sesame oil.

Preparation: Sauté cabbage and mushrooms in sesame oil, stir in soy sauce.

Day 5:

Breakfast: Baked Pears with Walnuts

Ingredients: Ripe pears, walnuts, cinnamon, honey (optional).

Preparation: Place pears on a baking sheet, sprinkle with walnuts and cinnamon; drizzle with honey if desired.

Lunch: Spinach and Artichoke Stuffed Chicken

Ingredients: Boneless, skinless chicken breasts, spinach, artichoke hearts, Parmesan cheese.

Preparation: Mix spinach, artichoke, and Parmesan; stuff into chicken, bake until cooked through.

Dinner: Sesame Ginger Salmon Patties

Ingredients: Canned salmon, soy sauce, sesame oil, fresh ginger.

Preparation: Combine salmon, soy sauce, sesame oil, and ginger; form into patties, pan-fry until golden.

Day 6:

Breakfast: Cucumber Noodle Salad with Mint

Ingredients: Cucumbers, cherry tomatoes, fresh mint, olive oil.

Preparation: Toss cucumber noodles, tomatoes, and mint with olive oil.

Lunch: Lemon Herb Roasted Veggies

Ingredients: Mixed vegetables, olive oil, fresh lemon juice, dried herbs (rosemary, thyme).

Preparation: Toss vegetables in olive oil, lemon juice, and herbs; roast until golden.

Dinner: Blueberry Chia Seed Pudding

Ingredients: Almond milk, chia seeds, blueberries, vanilla extract.

Preparation: Mix almond milk, chia seeds, blueberries, and vanilla; refrigerate until pudding-like consistency.

Day 7:

Breakfast: Stuffed Bell Peppers with Turkey and Quinoa

Ingredients: Bell peppers, cooked quinoa, lean ground turkey, tomato sauce.

Preparation: Mix quinoa, turkey, and tomato sauce; stuff into peppers, bake until tender.

Lunch: Coconut Almond Energy Bites

Ingredients: Shredded coconut, almond butter, honey, vanilla extract.

Preparation: Combine coconut, almond butter, honey, and vanilla; shape into small bites, refrigerate until firm.

Dinner: Your choice from the week's recipes – mix and match for variety!

CONCLUSION

The Sugar Detox Cookbook for Seniors is a guiding light on the path to better health. Through seven days of savory inquiry, this culinary guide has not only provided recipes but also served as a catalyst for transformation.

It challenges the narrative around elders and nutrition, demonstrating that every meal is an opportunity for vitality.

As the final page is turned, the cookbook leaves a legacy of increased vitality, resilience, and joy. Seniors, equipped with information and a variety of delicious dishes, may now enjoy life's sweetness without the dangerous embrace of refined sweets.

The Sugar Detox Cookbook is more than just a collection of recipes; it's a manifesto proclaiming that age is no barrier to a vibrant, health-conscious lifestyle. It demonstrates that, with the correct ingredients and perspective, seniors can enjoy the good things in life without sacrificing anything.

Happy cooking!

<u>Contact me here</u>

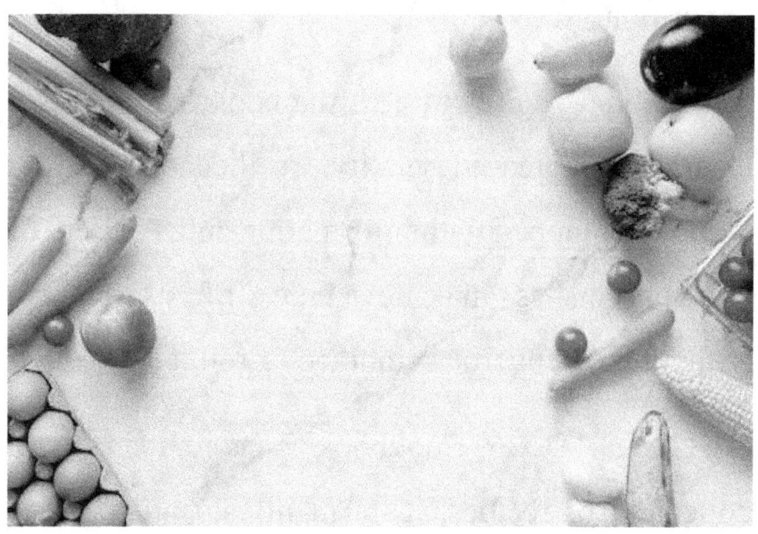